love

I AM...

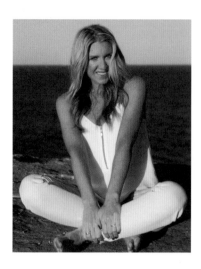

Danielle Wright grew up in Evergreen, a small mountain town just outside of Denver, Colorado. She went to school in both Colorado and Australia, and after graduating from Kansas University with a BA in Journalism, she began her advertising career in San Francisco then moved permanently to Australia.

Danielle met Mr. Wright in 1999 and they married in 2002. A few years later they became parents to two beautiful boys, Evan and Ben.

She ran a successful advertising agency for 12 years, and after deciding to move on, found her passion not only for art and writing, but for *life*.

This led her down a path of having a more loving, joyful, calm and forgiving state of mind. Through her own transformation, *Sleepy Magic* was born and is now an integral part of her family's life. She felt compelled to share her experience with like-minded parents so they can create their own special magic with their children.

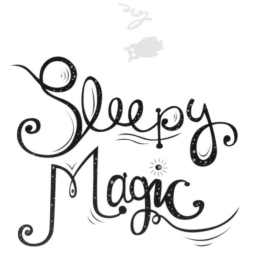

Sleepy Magic

A magical step-by-step
night-time ritual for
calm, connected and
conscious children

Written by Danielle Wright

Published by Feather Bound Publishing
PO Box 232, Waverley NSW 2024

Published 2014
Printed in China on behalf of the Opus Group

Cover and inside illustrations by Ina Kuehfuss

Photography by Lauren Callaghan

Book design by Denise Ayre

Every reasonable effort has been made to contact copyright holders of material reproduced in this book. If any have inadvertently been overlooked, the publishers would be glad to hear from them and make good in future editions any errors or omissions brought to their attention.

Quotes cited from the website *www.brainyquote.com*

www.daniellewright.com.au

National Library of Australia Cataloguing-in-Publication entry

Creator:	Wright, Danielle, author.
Title:	Sleepy Magic / Danielle Wright.
ISBN:	9780994180407 (hardback)
Target Audience:	For parents
Subjects:	Meditation for children.
	Parenting.
	Child rearing.
Dewey Number:	158.12083

For my three bears

Contents

You can find magic
wherever you look.
Sit back and relax
all you need is a book.

–Dr. Seuss

What's special about Sleepy Magic?

It's not by chance that you have picked up this book. It found you!

If one or all scenarios addressed within resonate with you, then the magic contained on these pages will make a difference in you, in your child and hopefully out in the wider world. If we as parents are calm, connected and conscious, it will empower our children to be the same.

Scenario #1
Solve Sleepless Nights

Are you reading this with your eyes half shut and hair in a tizz because you were up five times last night? (And the night before?) Come to think of it, you haven't had a decent night's sleep in days, weeks, months, even years. Ever since your sweet little angels decided that night-time was their playtime, they have become your sleepless nightmare.

Well, grab an espresso and perk up, because what you're about to read will change your life and your child's. Okay, a bit dramatic! But it will help your child sleep and in return you receive the ultimate pleasure. Sleep.

Do you want to have a calm, present and relaxed child at bedtime? Well, believe that you can! Within the first few minutes of the Sleepy Magic Meditation, you will see the calming effect. And after you are done, more often than not, you shouldn't hear a peep until morning.

Scenario #2
More Connection

Let's say your bub is a dream at sleep time. *Yes*! One battle you have overcome as a parent. However, are you a working or super busy parent struggling to find time to connect? I mean a soulful bond with your child, not just kicking a football around, playing dolls or reading a night-time story? Even though these times are definitely important too, don't you also want to create special time in our crazy world to completely focus on your child? And in return, your child will love every second of that attention.

With Sleepy Magic Meditation, not only will you make time to connect with each other, it will give your child space in their own mind to connect to their brilliance. It's possible! Each night you do the Sleepy Magic Meditation, you create a special ritual that connects you both emotionally and spiritually. This is about quality time.

Scenario #3
Nurture Stillness and Inner Harmony

Are you yourself into meditation, yoga, green juice, and feeling pretty good about how you treat your body, mind and spirit? Have you tapped into your own spiritual path?

However, your child refuses to eat anything but chicken nuggets, is crazy in love with the iPad or iPhone, and won't sit still for two minutes, let alone you trying to teach him or her to meditate. *Ha*! *Meditate*? You know for sure this would plain bore the pants off of them.

This is the beauty of Sleepy Magic Meditation. You are feeding them this good stuff without them realising it's the good stuff. The real good stuff. The stuff it takes some of us, including moi, half our lives to figure out.

Do you want to give your child a greater sense of themselves? Do you want to reinforce positive life habits? Teaching them to be calm, feel connection and become conscious at a young age is a wonderful gift. A lifetime gift you can give them. Yes, they are intuitive already. Certainly, children are naturally more connected and conscious. For some like myself though, we can disconnect while going through our teenage years and it takes years of work to get back to the heart of ourselves.

Give them the tools to ground themselves, know themselves and feel in control of their feelings right now.

Tried and True

If any of this rings true for you and your little one, then this just might be the magic you're looking for. I am not a meditation guru or yogi. I don't claim to be a sleeping expert. I'm a mum of two young boys and have been blessed to experience all of this with both of them. I'm truly passionate about this technique because it works.

Tried and tested by real families...

Mary, mother of three daughters aged 6, 7 and 9 had this to say about their Sleepy Magic experience:

"Sleepy Magic is a twinkling little gem. It is a beautiful bonding night-time ritual for my daughters and me. The stories we make up together become more magical and more exciting every time we do it. But Sleepy Magic has given them much more than that; it has introduced them to their inner voice and the realisation that strength, gentleness and happiness comes from within. What an incredible gift to give to every little girl."

Shared with like-minded parents who want to connect on a deeper level with their children...

Denise, mother of one daughter aged 7 said:

"I used the Sleepy Magic technique with my daughter Liv and since then she requests it every night. It has become our bedtime ritual - a beautiful 10 minutes of togetherness before she falls asleep. It calms us both down from our day. It focuses on the three special qualities we possess. And most importantly it gives us a mother/daughter tradition that I feel will be passed down to her children one day."

You are shaping your child's world.

As parents, we know it's extremely important for us to feed, shelter, educate, protect and love our little ones. But what about tending to their soul, their spirit, their inner being, or whatever you like to call this energy?

This guide is a beautiful and easy way to introduce meditation and affirmations into your children's lives. It will open their hearts to find their own joy lies within.

And the fantastic upside? Everyone in the house gets some well-deserved sleep!

At the end of the day, the most
overwhelming key to a child's success is
the positive involvement of parents.
– Jane D. Hull

That is the real spiritual awakening,
when something emerges from within
you that is deeper than who you thought
you were. So, the person is still there,
but one could almost say that something more
powerful shines through the person.
– Eckhart Tolle

A bit of
background

It's never too late to change your life. In fact, whether you realise it or not, each time you wake in the morning you have a choice to change yourself. You can embrace the new possibilities or stay in your old patterns.

The principles I discuss in this book are for you *and* your children. They may be completely new to you. They may not. I have taken well-known principles and structured them into an easy-to-understand guide for you to use to open yourself to the everyday possibilities of change.

These same principles are sprinkled throughout the Sleepy Magic Meditation too. When I first started this with my children, trust me, I had no idea what an impact it would make on my life. Not to mention their lives. My experience has continued expanding as this book and the meditations in it took shape. And it will keep on doing so each and every day.

It took what I considered my mid-life crisis to finally ignite my authentic self and create the life I deserve. I want to share my experience so that you can find your inner light and start fanning your own flames without having to crash and burn first.

A few years ago, I was cruising through life and (from the outside) had it all. But on the inside something was amiss. All of these wonderful things I had externally were not making me happy anymore. Not only was I fearful and stressed about keeping up as a good mum, wife and business owner, but the guilt was crushing. And in not wanting to fail others, I was failing myself. Like many supermums, I was physically, emotionally and mentally burnt out and numbing out.

In the beginning of 2012, it all came to a head. I knew about positive energy and the Law of Attraction thanks to Oprah and reading *The Secret*. However, I was doing the opposite and manifesting major negative events out of sheer fear and stress. Well, it wasn't pretty. I was getting uglier on the inside by the minute. This was not only affecting me, but my relationship with my husband, my children, my creativity, my self-worth. The lot. I had always been the strong, assertive, risk-taking, happy-go-lucky, fun one. Instead, I felt weak, unstable, worried, in a constant state of stress. My thoughts were endlessly on repeat about the past or the future. I was consistently saying yes to people and situations that only created feelings of resentment within me.

Life was sending me clear messages that I needed to change. First it was a whisper. Then it was a poke. And then there were some major slaps. It didn't let up for 6 months. But finally my advertising agency of 12 years, my first baby, had to suddenly and unexpectedly shut its doors. That happening was the rock to the head.

The transformation to finding my authentic self began with a search for my light again. I realised I needed help beyond my family and friends. I needed some major self-care. A friend advised me to see an amazing kinesiologist/neuro-trainer named Deborah Beers (www.deborahbeers.com). Not only did she help me heal myself into a calmer, connected, and certainly more conscious being, but she was there at the most emotional, stressful and heartbreaking time, when my business ceased to exist. I was more prepared to handle it and see the beautiful blue skies beyond the situation. It was my chance to change my life and do it completely on my terms.

Most importantly, I knew how I wanted to feel inside from that moment on; that was to be fab, fulfilled, and excited. And when most of the dust had settled, I realised I hadn't had a mid-life crisis at all. I'd had a mid-life *a w a k e n i n g*.

Now, you may be wondering what a kinesiologist is. Deborah specialises in gently releasing your mental, emotional and physical patterns and habits that block you from living the life you deserve. According to Deborah, kinesiology/neuro-training assists the brain to adapt more easily and to find the most positive change in all circumstances.

For me, she removed energy that has been stored in my body from childhood experiences. I had formed patterns of behaviour (mainly triggered by stress and issues of self-worth) in my adult life around these experiences or traumas. One of these was a near-death experience when I was two-and-a-half years old when a neighbour gave me a peanut butter cookie and I had a full-blown anaphylactic reaction. By the grace of the Universe, my grandfather was baby sitting me that day. Being a doctor, he had his medical bag with him and knew I had gone into anaphylactic shock. Of course, in those days, a nut allergy was very rare. I only vaguely remember the incident, but my body has stored that trauma somehow and held on to the fear for 40 years. For all that time, I had fear-based reactions to certain situations because of that moment in my young life. Go figure!

After the kinesiology sessions and new tools that Deb had given me, I felt massive healing occur. I noticed that I started to grow in a more healthy, less stressful way. And I wanted more of those feelings.

I started to meditate, which at first was quite difficult, since I had created such an obscenely busy life and felt much guilt for putting myself first. My mind was also all over the shop! How could I possibly switch it off?

I began with guided meditation and then yoga, until something clicked within and it became peaceful and blissful to just sit in silence. I can now very happily meditate for more extended periods of time. I crave my meditations because I am actually more productive afterwards. And not only do I feel the healing benefits, but also a lot of inspiration and insight comes to me while I am at peace.

While peacing out instead of numbing out, I got very curious about this notion that we are spiritual beings having a human experience, not the other way around. I became a sponge for spiritual knowledge and read Eckhart Tolle, Wayne Dyer, Louise Hay, Doreen Virtue, Cheryl Richardson and works by so many other amazing people. With this new knowledge, I started to practice being present. Personally, I had to practice being in the now because I was so concerned and worried with the past or future that my mind would hold on to events or create future scenarios that most likely wouldn't happen. It was and is a waste of my energy. All that is important is right *now*.

The next piece of my curiosity puzzle was discovered at Christmas time in 2013. I decided that, instead of having a New Year's Resolution, I picked one word of how I wanted to feel this next year and live my life to that word. My word was *passionate*.

I now make my daily decision to feel this way, from work, to play, to being with my husband and children. In fact, a month later I came across a wonderful woman named Danielle LaPorte who created a book called The Desire Map, which is all about finding your Core Desired Feelings, then each day living and breathing by them. It has absolutely changed my life. I worked out that I want to feel exquisite, inspired, connected and joyful every day. I even do the mundane grocery shopping with these feelings in mind - I stick on my headphones, listen to my favourite playlist, and bop my way down the aisle with a smile on my face. Some people look at me funny, but more times than not they smile back at me!

Through all of this, I became softer and more compassionate to my husband, my sons, my family, friends, strangers and most importantly myself. Yes, I am still practicing not beating myself up when I react to my triggers. Now instead of using a whip, I use a feather boa... I just let go a lot more easily.

Within the mix of all this life-changing stuff, Sleepy Magic was born. Almost a year into my transformation, I attended a course that my kinesiologist Deborah teaches called "Living Life Passionately". By using practical processes and guided meditations in her two-day workshop, I let go of burdens from my past and unlocked key desires to my present and future. I was so pumped and inspired by the entire process that I went home that night and performed a mini-meditation on our son Evan, who had just turned 7 at the time. Some parts of the meditation were taken from Deborah's teachings and the rest were inspired through me. Eventually, it became a combination of both our work which I have footnoted in the book.

I couldn't believe how receptive, calm and open Evan was to meditation.

Since then, it has transformed and progressed into a wonderful ritual that together we coined Sleepy Magic. He asks for it every night without fail. It worked so well that I started to do it for our very active 3 year old, Ben. *Et voilà*, the magic worked on his restless age as well.

Bedtime is now a calm, loving, sweet dream space for our entire household. Here, I share my learnings and Sleepy Magic meditation with the world, so that you and your family can experience the magic also.

Nothing is more important than
reconnecting with your bliss.
Nothing is as rich.
Nothing is more real.
– Deepak Chopra

Creating the life you love

Life is a personal journey. Like fingerprints, it is unique to each one of us. In my own journey, I have started to practice five important lessons that have led me down a path of a less stressful and more joyful existence. For us to teach our children mindfulness, we need to teach ourselves to be more mindful. I want to stress that you absolutely do not have to do any of the following practices yourself to see the benefits that Sleepy Magic has on your children if your main goal is for them to have a routine to sleep. However, if something resonates, take the time to explore it and see for yourself if you feel a difference.

There are five steps to what I call the *Cycle of SELF*. Each step relates to the other. Once you tap into them, you can feel the change within.

Now, you might have the perception that it takes hard work to get the life you deserve or that your dream is somewhere in the future. Have you ever used the phrase "I'll be happy when this happens" or "I will be successful when I have this"? Well, sure. It's all fine to think that. Have you then felt happy or successful reaching your goal, but the feeling dissipates days, hours, or just seconds later? Even worse, it may be a let down when you reach your goal and you don't feel that high of being happy or successful at all. So you go straight back to chasing down the next big achievement.

By practicing the Cycle of SELF, you can have the feelings you seek in those moments, because you are living in the moment! And the more you practice, the better you feel; the better you feel, the more you practice. Don't you want to be high on life a lot more of the time? You don't have to wait. The power is already yours. And theirs. This is a major point in Sleepy Magic. The meditation is an introduction to your child practicing the Cycle of SELF for them to grow from the inside out.

SELF stands for Source Energising your Life Force. When I refer to SELF, it means your Source (you may refer it as your soul, Spirit, inner being, the Universe, Divine, unconditional love) that Energises (grows, empowers, reinforces) your Life Force (your self-worth and the energy tied to that self-worth, either positive or negative) that you project out in the world.

Personally, I visualise and feel my Source as a warm gold light, which I use in Sleepy Magic. It is alive in the Solar Plexus which is located underneath the rib cage in the centre of the body. The Solar Plexus is one of our 7 Chakras. (The Chakras are covered in further detail later.)

As you can see from the image, your Authentic SELF is in the middle, sitting in a gold circle. As you start practicing the 5 Cs, your gold light expands and gets stronger. The 5 Cs are CALM, CONNECT, CONSCIOUS, CORE DESIRES, and CREATE. And the ideal is to practice these 5 Cs until that gold light becomes so illuminated that it expands outside your body; that is when people notice and feel your light.

Think of a time when a person walked in the room and had something about them that was so magnetising. You couldn't put your finger on it. From the outside, they may not be the prettiest, smartest or the most successful, but they glowed. How pretty, smart and successful is that? They have tapped into their Source and it's Energising their Life Force. It's making their gold light so bright that you sense it. Now, I don't know if I have reached the magnetising point, but recently a good friend who has been witnessing the changes in my life over the past two years, asked me, "What is it? What are you doing? It's like you are drinking joy juice and I want to know how I can get some?"

Let me explain the 5 Cs and how they get me juiced up on joy.

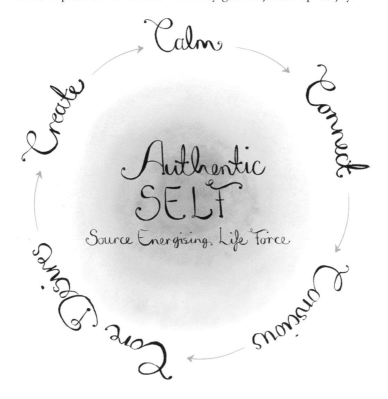

The 5 Cs and their relation to SELF

1. Calm

If you want to create the life you deserve, the first step is to CALM down. This means making time to care for your SELF. This is your time to let it go, learn and be SELFish. Yes, taking time for you is as necessary as breathing. If you don't take time for you, you are not being your optimal best for you or for your children. Through practices of meditation (even for five minutes a day), yoga, using the head-holding and breathing technique (refer to page 29), you will relieve stress and come back to a better state of mind. Even something as simple as taking a walk in nature, dancing, singing, being creative by painting or drawing will shift and release negative/ disruptive energy and you begin to heal.

To maximise SELF-care, you can explore and seek alternative therapies such as reiki, kinesiology, acupressure, acupuncture and reflexology, releasing blocked energy. Your body stores energy from past experiences even as far back as being in the womb. When you unblock these energies, it breaks patterns that you may or may not know you are doing or experiencing in adulthood. This is a very personal experience so find what works for you.

2. Connect

The moment you feel CALMer, your energy shifts and you become CONNECTed and grounded. You tap into Mother Earth, to community or relationships, and most importantly to your Source.

My greatest inspiration comes from tapping into my Source. For me, when I am CALM by walking in nature or in meditation, my Source presents me with creative ideas. For instance, this entire concept of the Cycle of SELF was handed to me through one of the most powerful and amazing meditations I have experienced to date. It flashed in front of my mind so very clearly. And at the time I wasn't thinking; just being. I was that CONNECTed to my Source, the image of the diagram flashed in my mind's eye and it literally brought tears to my eyes. It made perfect sense.

To feel CONNECTed to SELF, try waking up each day (you are naturally calm already at this time) and writing down three things you are grateful for. When you are grateful, the negative elements of your life don't seem as big or important.

Another great tool is to repeat positive affirmations three times to yourself. You will be amazed how different you feel about yourself when you repeat three little words of "I am strong", "I am happy", "I am incredible" etc. Your SELF will start to glow even more and your heart will become lighter.

Another major part of CONNECTing is forgiveness. Once you let go of old wounds, situations, people and truly forgive them, you can forgive yourself and be free. You do not have to be friends, stay friends or even see people again to forgive them, but you can decide to move on. Once you find the space in your heart to let go, a whole new world will open.

3. Conscious

Living in the now is a key part of having the life you are meant to have.

The past is exactly that, the past... If your mind is consistently revisiting memories, you are not living in the present. If you are consistently worried about the future or creating scenarios in your mind that may or may not even happen (it's almost always the latter), you are not living now. The only moment that counts is this one.

Being CONSCIOUS takes practice because we are in the habit of living in the past and future, but if you are practicing being CALM and CONNECTed, this is the natural next step. You will begin to catch your mind in a spin and start to manage what you think. It is impossible to stop all thought unless you are a monk, but it is possible to control and shift the thoughts by focusing on what you are doing. You will begin to feel unconditional love and non-judgement of yourself and others.

The head-holding and breathing technique which is explained on page 29 is fantastic for snapping you into being present and centred.

4. Core desires

Aha! Now that your mind is CALM, CONNECTED and CONSCIOUS, this gives you space to focus on your CORE DESIRES. These are the ultimate feelings you want to have.

Just like having a choice in what you are thinking, you also have a choice in how you are feeling. Happiness, joy, freedom, abundance, health, alertness, bravery, pleasure, creativity... the list is endless. It is completely up to you. Yes, life will always throw you curve balls and sometimes it feels awful, scary and painful, but these feelings are temporary and you control how long you hold onto them.

It's like bungy-jumping (so I am told). You feel terrified, but once you jump and take that risk, you release the fear and within seconds you are elated and feel *alive*!

You can also release a feeling. Feel it, sit in it and then release it because the situation has now become part of the past and you can refocus on your CORE DESIRES once again. Remember, no person, place or situation can control how you feel. Feelings are our road map to navigating what we truly want. Listen to them, then let yourself be free.

Set an intention of how you are going to feel when you wake up. Say yes to everything that makes you feel that way and say no (in the nicest possible way) to any person, place or situation that doesn't align with those CORE DESIRES. How do you want to feel right *now*? Choose it and stick to it.

5. Create

Now it's all starting to come together. You are directing your life down the path you want. Thinking and feeling how you want. You are grounded, centred and lighter in your heart. To put it simply, it's the Law of Attraction and what you focus on grows. You want that growth to be positive, to be SELF-confident, SELF-assured, SELF-empowered, SELF-improved and SELF-worthy.

The flip side is that the gold light can retract. If you are not CALM (in state of stress), not CONNECTed (isolated from others, from nature, from the divine), not CONSCIOUS (worried or your thoughts are on endless repeat), and you constantly dishonour your CORE DESIRES (saying yes to the things you don't want and those situations that create negative feelings and resentment), you will only invite in a life of misery and begin to numb out with all sorts of addictions. Your SELF is depleted. You have low SELF-esteem, high SELF-doubt, and more SELF-criticism, which leads you to SELF-destruct.

The best way I can describe what I have found through this process is that I have more peaceful space in my mind. Instead of my mind full of clutter and useless garbage, I now have more space to concentrate on the thoughts/feelings/things/people that matter the most to me.

The Cycle of SELF is exactly that: an infinite cycle always in motion forward. Once you notice that the energy on the inside is manifesting new experiences on the outside, you will start to feel elevated emotions of empowerment, strength, love, joy and gratitude. That new, better, wonderful energy will be the momentum you need to keep repeating the steps in the cycle. Remember, to have the joy juice, you take baby steps. You can't expect it to happen overnight but it will happen. You will continue to reclaim your power, and so your SELF.

Ultimately, you are SELF-seeking and creating the life you deserve!

Just imagine becoming the way you used to be as a very
young child, before you understood the meaning of any
word, before opinions took over your mind. The real you
is loving, joyful, and free. The real you is just like a flower,
just like the wind, just like the ocean, just like the sun.
– Miguel Angel Ruiz

What you need to know before you start

In the next sections, I explain in depth the 5 steps to Sleepy Magic. Don't panic about how much text there is to read; the more you do it, the easier it becomes. Like your own journey, it will become unique for you and your child.

The 5 steps are:

Step 1 - Pick 7 tabs from the Sleepy Magic box (optional)

Step 2 - Ask the question "What are you proud of today?"

Step 3 - Head-hold and breathing technique

Step 4 - Example Story of the Rainbow Bears

Step 5 - Putting a filter on your child's Chakras/energy

I have included two extra stories in the back of this book for you to try, but once you get the essential repetitive structure of the meditation story, you can adapt the places, objects, people, animals to what your child likes. Dinosaurs, ballet, sports, superheroes, princesses and fairies, absolutely anything your child's heart desires. I have used magical creatures, car races, volcanoes, planes and parachutes, characters like Super Mario and Pikachu, Santa and even Minecraft. My kids now set challenges and pick obscure objects or scenarios to see if I can come up with another story. The most recent one was Benny skateboarding over sharks. Love the imagination!

Because the meditation is repetitive and easy to follow, in their eyes, I have become the smartest mum in the world. Be as creative as you want and you will find your child will request certain scenarios he or she loves.

This book is a guide to tap into your imagination and help your children grow from the inside out. Who wouldn't want to strengthen the bond with their child? Not only will you be teaching them that they are spiritually safe, but that they have the power to be happy, healthy and in control of their internal path by building positivity and self-esteem.

Take note, it's important to finish the meditation even if your child falls asleep (*yay*!) because what you say will be embedded into their subconscious. Play soft meditation music if you want. Remember it's about creating your special ritual. Add or subtract whatever feels right to you.

You might feel awkward reading and want to try to sound natural. I can guarantee your children will not care if you don't do it perfectly! They are just happy to have you. I promise it will become more natural as time goes on and you will have more confidence in your delivery.

I suggest you familiarise yourself with the steps and repeat the same story to your child over a few nights. Once you are comfortable with the structure, feel free to mix it up. Use one of the stories outlined later in this book or unleash your wonderful imagination. Go crazy! It's your ritual and you know your child best. If you need help or just want to see how this works, watch the demo video of our ritual on *http://www.daniellewright.com.au/demo-meditation-video* and use password: love&light

What in the world is a Chakra?

You might be wondering what step 5 is all about.

As I have previously discussed, we have energy that is radiating from us. We control what sort of energy we feel inside and project out, whether that is positive (joy juice!) or negative.

There are 7 main points (or energy centres) located in the body that are related to different aspects of our lives like wealth, love, health, communication, creativity and our connection to the spirituality. These are called Chakras. It is vital to keep the Chakras clear and healthy so you can feel as good as possible. If we hold on to negative thoughts, the Chakras can become dull, dirty and unbalanced. The energy can become lethargic and sometimes turn to illness. Each one is a different colour of the rainbow and looks like a spinning funnel or waterspout pushing the energy around our body. This is where meditation comes in.

In Sleepy Magic, you are working with the Chakra colours to keep them healthy and bright.

I focus mainly on the Solar Plexus Chakra using affirmation. This is the Chakra that empowers your child's SELF-worth. Even though they cannot control external life itself, working with Chakras teaches them they have the ultimate power to grow their SELF-worth. This step is just simply putting a protective filter on your child's Chakras so it keeps other people's energy out and theirs in. I keep the Crown Chakra (located at the very top of the head) and the Base Chakra (located at the base of the spine in the tailbone area) open because you draw energy and inspiration from the Universe through your Crown Chakra down through each Chakra in the body out through the Base Chakra and into the earth which grounds the ideas and goals.

For information on Chakras, I suggest a book called *Chakras for Beginners: How to Balance, Strengthen Aura and Radiate Energy* by Victoria Lane. For an interesting take on how Chakras affect your life, there is also a book called *Defying Gravity* by Caroline Myss. On page 24 is a simple explanation and illustration of which colour correlates to which Chakra and what each Chakra represents.

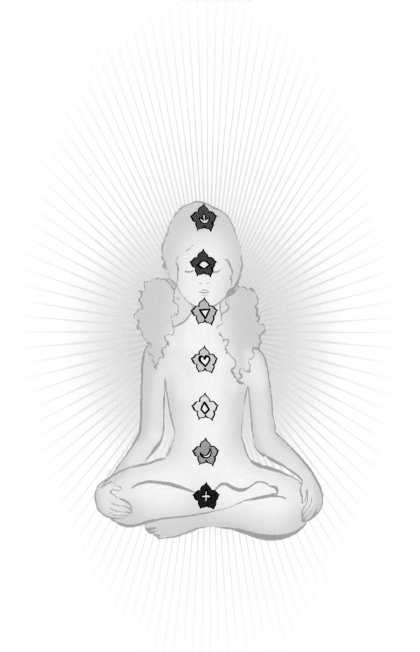

*When you get to a place where you understand that love
and belonging, your worthiness, is a birthright and not
something you have to earn, anything is possible.*
– Brene Brown

All Chakras are in the front and the back of the body.

Base Chakra (red) - Location: Base of the spine in the tailbone area. Represents our foundation (survival needs) and the feeling of being grounded. Emotional issues: security and vitality.

Creative Chakra (orange) - Location: Lower abdomen, about two inches below the belly button. The centre for expressing creativity, connection and ability to accept others and new experiences. Emotional issues: Creativity, wellbeing and feeling compassion.

Solar Plexus Chakra (yellow) - Location: Underneath the rib cage in the centre of the body. Ability to be confident and in control of our lives. Where we manifest our desires and intentions. Emotional issues: Self-worth, confidence and sense of belonging.

Heart Chakra (green) - Location: Centre of the chest. Ability to love and create a loving life. Emotional issues: Unconditional love, forgiveness, social identity.

Throat Chakra (blue) - Location: Throat. Ability to communicate. Emotional issues: Communication and self-expression.

Third Eye Chakra (indigo) - Location: Centre of the forehead between the eyes. Ability to focus on and see the big picture. Emotional issues: Intuition, imagination, insight, and self-knowledge.

Crown Chakra (violet) - Location: The very top of the head. Ability to be fully connected spiritually. Emotional issues: Inner and outer beauty, our connection to spirituality, integration of the whole.

Today you are you!
That is truer than true!
There is no one alive who is you-er than you!
– Dr. Seuss

5 steps
to Sleepy Magic

Step 1: Sleepy Magic container (optional)

In the back of this book are the "I am..." affirmation tabs that you can use in your ritual. Cut out the tabs and put them in a box, tin or bag. Only cut out and use tabs you think are age-appropriate or will resonate with your child.

We painted our little box gold and put gold sparkles on it. Judy, a mother of two girls, said that her 5-year-old Charlotte chose to use her special Disney princess bucket to keep her tabs in. Be as creative as you want or use something you know your child will like.

If you do use the tabs in the meditation, remember to have your child give the tabs back to you once they pick them so you can read the tabs. You want them to be absorbed by your voice not fiddling with pieces of paper or reading the affirmations themselves. Their eyes should be shut during the meditation.

The affirmations are a major part of Sleepy Magic, but using the tabs and box idea is completely optional. By all means wing it and make up your own "I am" or use pages 55 and 57 as a quick reference. Some examples are: I am special, I am helpful, I am smart, I am loving... etc.

I suggest you come up with the affirmations as you do the meditation to begin with because you want your child to calm, connect and become conscious in the meditation. However, once you have your method down, your child might state their own "I am..." affirmation. Brilliant, go with it. My youngest son will occasionally say one or two "I am..." affirmations during the meditation that he feels strongly about and wants to be.

For ebook users or if you do not want to cut up this beautiful book you can visit *http://www.daniellewright.com.au/affirmation-tabs* and use password: iam to download a pdf of the "I am..." affirmations or simply hand write them or use your computer.

Once your child is nestled in bed, ask them to pick 7 tabs and hand them to you.

Step 2: Ask the question "What are you proud of today?"

The more you praise and celebrate your life,
the more there is in life to celebrate.
– Oprah Winfrey

In a soft voice ask them what they are proud of for the day. Then you respond with what you are proud of doing. This can be as simple as going to school, helping with the dishes, hugging a sibling, being kind to a friend or much grander acts of kindness and consideration. Even go as far as asking them how it made them feel.

Ask them to give themselves a hug and give yourself one too. This affirms their actions, ingrains a greater sense of SELF and will fill both your hearts with pride. And who doesn't like hugs? They are extremely healing.

This is a great way to boost their self-esteem, open communication and be in touch with what makes them tick. You find out very quickly whether or not you are leading by example by your own answers. And you may be surprised how much or little you are proud of yourself for doing each day. Remember it's not about the big stuff like Mummy won a promotion or Daddy made lots of money which is wonderful for you. It's about showing kindness to others like praising a co-worker or friend, telling a sales lady you think her necklace is beautiful, or maybe you just smiled your way down the street at 10 strangers. These tiny acts are the ones that light up our hearts because you are making someone else's moment special and that's truly something to be proud of.

Another question you can ask instead is "What are you grateful for today?" This is also a lovely way to engage your child with what is important in life to them. By being grateful they can significantly change how they feel about their life. It quickly puts everything into perspective.

Step 3: Head-hold and breathing exercise

Breathing is central to every aspect of meditation training. It's a wonderful place to focus in training the mind to be calm and concentrated.

– Jon Kabat-Zinn

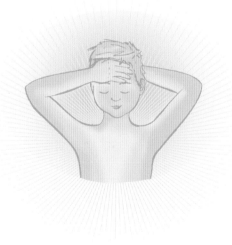

This step is essential for calming and preparing your child for Sleepy Magic and sleep. If they are sitting up, have them lie on their back and put one hand on the bumpy bit on the back of their head and one hand on their forehead as shown in the diagram.

Tell them to close their eyes. Say "breathe in" (now count silently for 4). Then say "hold" (and count silently for 2). Next say "breathe out" (and count silently for 4).

Repeat until you notice your child relaxing. It takes 9 repetitions.

I tend to use my hand and gently stroke them from their throats to their bellies with each in and out breathe. Your child may be very ticklish and this might be distracting if you touch them.

When nice and relaxed, ask your little one to put their arms by their side palms facing up.

Since my boys and I have been doing Sleepy Magic for a long time now, they will lay on their sides or back. Remember, there is no wrong way to do this. If they are more comfortable in a different position, by all means let them lie that way.

This breathing technique is one of the handiest tricks Deborah Beers has taught me about alleviating stress and making you instantly present. As I mentioned in the 5 Cs, this is a wonderful way to CALM, CONNECT and become CONSCIOUS all at once.

practice this yourself and you will be surprised how it helps with your own meditation, a sleepless night, dealing with a cranky boss or a downright horrid person and most of all the dreaded witching hour each night that seems to last a lot longer than an hour! By the 3rd or 4th breath, you will feel your stress level drop. You will also regain clarity over a situation. It is a technique I use almost daily and I have even seen my son do it before a running race... and he won!

Please check out the demo video on how to do the head-holding and breathing technique on *http://www.daniellewright.com.au/breathing-technique-video* and use password: letgo

Step 4: Story of the Little Rainbow Bears

There are no rules of architecture for a castle in the clouds.

– Gilbert K. Chesterton

The red text is the meditation you softly say to your child after he or she is calm and relaxed. You can lightly stroke their forehead, throat and tummy at the same time if your child isn't too ticklish or gets too distracted.

The black text is my direction for you. I have included this story and two others from page 37 without direction.

Your child's eyes should be closed.

Now onto the story...

"I want you to think of any yucky things people said or did to you today, or even things you did that you don't feel so good about. Imagine those yucky things like weeds sprouting inside you. Do you see them in your mind *(place your hand on their forehead)*, or in your heart *(place your hand on their heart)*, or in your tummy *(place your hand on their tummy)*? I want you to pluck all those ugly weeds and throw them in the bin. Now take a stick of dynamite, light it and throw that in the bin. And kaboom! *(Children love noises so feel free to express your best blowing up sounds!)* All the yucky weeds are blown up, gone forever.

Now you take my hand and we walk into a beautiful forest. We come across a huge tree with a big door in the middle. We knock on the door and it opens. Inside, we see seven colourful bears sitting around a table smiling and laughing. They ask us to sit with them.

The red bear hands you a pot of red honey. You lick the honey and it forms a red ray from a rainbow that slides down your throat. As it goes down, you say I am... *(Now read the first tab in your hand, eg. happy)*.

I am happy, I am happy, I am happy. Say it three times in your head and the red ray turns to a gold seed right here. *(Touch your child under their rib cage in the centre of their body; this is the solar plexus, which is the centre of their being.)*

The orange bear hands you a pot of orange honey. You lick the honey and it forms an orange ray from a rainbow that slides down your throat. As it goes down, you say I am... *(Now read the next tab in your hand)*.

I am..., I am..., I am... Say it three times in your head and then the orange ray turns to a gold seed right here. *(Touch the solar plexus)*.

The yellow bear passes you the pot of yellow honey. You lick the honey and it forms a yellow ray from a rainbow that slides down your throat. As it goes down, you say I am... *(Read the next tab in your hand)*.

I am..., I am..., I am... Say it three times in your head and the yellow ray turns to a gold seed right here. *(Touch the solar plexus)*.

The green bear passes you the pot of green honey. You lick the honey and it forms a green ray from a rainbow that slides down your throat. As it goes down, you say I am... *(Read the next tab in your hand)*.

I am..., I am..., I am... Say it three times in your head and the green ray turns to a gold seed right here. *(Touch the solar plexus)*.

The blue bear passes you the pot of blue honey. You lick the honey and it forms a blue ray from a rainbow that slides down your throat. As it goes down, you say I am... *(Read the next tab in your hand)*.

I am..., I am..., I am... Say it three times in your head and the blue ray turns to a gold seed right here. *(Touch the solar plexus)*.

The indigo *(or dark blue)* bear passes you the pot of indigo honey. You lick the honey and it forms an indigo ray from a rainbow that slides down your throat. As it goes down, you say I am... *(Read the next tab in your hand)*.

I am..., I am..., I am... Say it three times in your head and the indigo ray turns to a gold seed right here. *(Touch the solar plexus)*.

The last bear is the violet *(or purple)* bear, who finally passes you the pot of violet honey. You lick the honey and it forms a violet ray from a rainbow that slides down your throat. As it goes down, you say I am... *(Read the next tab in your hand)*.

I am..., I am..., I am... Say it three times in your head and the violet ray turns to a gold seed right here. *(Touch the solar plexus)*.

Now you have seven magic seeds inside of you and to make them grow you have to pour gold light onto them. Only you have the power to do this. In the centre of your body, there is a gold light. It's right here *(touch the solar plexus again under the rib cage)*. Pour your gold light onto the seeds. Now look and feel the seeds grow into a gold plant with branches, vines, and gold flowers. It grows all the way to the tips of your toes, fingertips and top of your head. It gets bigger and brighter. It gets so big and bright it pops outside your body.

Now you're sitting in a gold bubble.[1] Suck the gold bubble onto the outside of your body.[2] It forms a gold suit. *(It could be gold armour, gold second skin, gold spacesuit or gold superhero suit).*[3] This gold suit keeps you spiritually safe and protected at all times. You will now have a beautiful sleep and wake up in the morning filled with happiness and ready for what the day brings.

Now I'll help you close your Chakras."

Step 5: Closing your child's Chakras/energy points

Self-worth comes from one thing
- thinking that you are worthy.
– Wayne Dyer

To close your child's Chakras, simply repeat the words below.

I touch my kids with my index and middle finger and make the motions down and across on each of their Chakra points for them to identify where they sit in the body.

"Imagine there is a window in the middle of your forehead. Shut the window, close the curtains.
There is a window in both of your ears. Shut the window, close the curtains.
There is a window in your throat. Shut the window, close the curtains.

And on the same spot on the back of your throat. Shut the window, close the curtains.

Now right on your heart, see the window? Shut the window, close the curtains.

And now on your back in the same spot. Shut the window, close the curtains.

On your solar plexus. Shut the window, close the curtains.

And on the same spot on your back. Shut the window, close the curtains.

Below your belly button. Shut the window, close the curtains.

And on the same spot on your back. Shut the window, close the curtains.[4]

Good night. Have wonderful dreams. I love you and I'm proud of you being you."

Of course if you want to add anything else, go ahead.

As you will see on my demo video, I have cut the words down since my sons are already accustomed to the ritual and visualise the process. I do not include "there is a window in the middle of your forehead" any longer.

Note above (1-4 Deborah Beers).

The 5 Steps

Step 1 - Pick 7 tabs from the Sleepy Magic box (optional)

Step 2 - Ask the question "What are you proud of today?"

Step 3 - Head-hold and breathing technique

Step 4 - Meditation Story

Step 5 - Putting a filter on your child's Chakras/energy

Words of encouragement

The child must know that he is a miracle, that since the beginning of the world there hasn't been, and until the end of the world there will not be, another child like him.
– Pablo Casals

The first few times you do Sleepy Magic, you might feel tongue-tied, believe you're not doing it right or fumble around trying to come up with ideas.

Trust me you can't mess it up. Your child will embrace it because they love you. In their eyes, you are their light. The more you practice, the more natural it will become.

Touching your child is really important for bonding and soothing, but some might find it very ticklish. I suggest occasionally placing your hand on their heart for tactile feedback.

You may have more than one child and be feeling very stretched for time. Feel free to do Sleepy Magic with both, or all three, four, or five of them at the same time in one bed. Then transfer the children to their own beds afterwards. My boys do have different bedtimes so I can make time for both. On the nights they have a sleepover together, we will do Sleepy Magic all together.

And of course, you can make it a routine every other night or in between other activities like reading.

A great way to reinforce the "I am..." affirmations is to discuss them the next day in the car on the way to school, day care or an outing. Before the boys jump out of the car for school, I touch the top of their heads and make a funny Star Trek "beam me up, Scotty" noise. Then I tell them I am covering them in gold light to form their suit. I ask what their "I am..." affirmation is for the day. They love this and ask for their gold bubble if I forget which is more times than not!

I have included a blank page for you to take down any notes, story ideas or other inspiration at the back of the book.

Please visit me at *www.daniellewright.com.au* to find out about the magic beyond this book. And while you are there, drop me a line. I would love to hear about your triumphs and personal stories.

Sleepy
Magic
stories

love

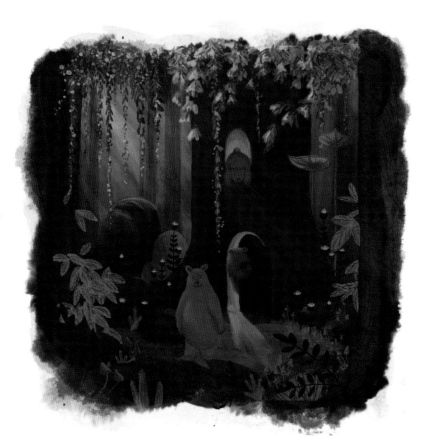

Story of the Little Rainbow Bears

"I want you to think of any yucky things people said or did to you today, or even things you did that you don't feel so good about. Imagine those yucky things like weeds sprouting inside you. Do you see them in your mind or in your heart or in your tummy? I want you to pluck all those ugly weeds and throw them in the bin. Now take a stick of dynamite, light it and throw that in the bin. And kaboom! All the yucky weeds are blown up, gone forever.

Now you take my hand and we walk into a beautiful forest. We come across a huge tree with a big door in the middle. We knock on the door and it opens. Inside, we see seven colourful bears sitting around a table smiling and laughing. They ask us to sit with them.

The red bear hands you a pot of red honey. You lick the honey and it forms a red ray from a rainbow that slides down your throat. As it goes down, you say I am...

I am..., I am..., I am... Say it three times in your head and the red ray turns to a gold seed right here.

The orange bear hands you a pot of orange honey. You lick the honey and it forms an orange ray from a rainbow that slides down your throat. As it goes down, you say I am...

I am..., I am..., I am... Say it three times in your head and then the orange ray turns to a gold seed right here.

The yellow bear passes you the pot of yellow honey. You lick the honey and it forms a yellow ray from a rainbow that slides down your throat. As it goes down, you say I am...

I am..., I am..., I am... Say it three times in your head and the yellow ray turns to a gold seed right here.

The green bear passes you the pot of green honey. You lick the honey and it forms a green ray from a rainbow that slides down your throat. As it goes down, you say I am...

I am..., I am..., I am... Say it three times in your head and the green ray turns to a gold seed right here.

The blue bear passes you the pot of blue honey. You lick the honey and it forms a blue ray from a rainbow that slides down your throat. As it goes down, you say I am...

I am..., I am..., I am... Say it three times in your head and the blue ray turns to a gold seed right here.

The indigo bear passes you the pot of indigo honey. You lick the honey and it forms an indigo ray from a rainbow that slides down your throat. As it goes down, you say I am...

I am..., I am..., I am... Say it three times in your head and the indigo ray turns to a gold seed right here.

The last bear is the violet bear, who finally passes you the pot of violet honey. You lick the honey and it forms a violet ray from a rainbow that slides down your throat. As it goes down, you say I am.....

I am..., I am..., I am... Say it three times in your head and the violet ray turns to a gold seed right here.

Now you have seven magic seeds inside of you and to make them grow you have to pour gold light onto them. Only you have the power to do this. In the centre of your body, there is a gold light. It's right here. Pour your gold light onto the seeds. Now look and feel the seeds grow into a gold plant with branches, vines, and gold flowers. It grows all the way to the tips of your toes, fingertips and top of your head. It gets bigger and brighter. It gets so big and bright it pops outside your body.

Now you're sitting in a gold bubble. Suck the gold bubble onto the outside of your body. It forms a gold suit. This gold suit keeps you spiritually safe and protected at all times. You will now have a beautiful sleep and wake up in the morning filled with happiness and ready for what the day brings.

Now I will help you close your Chakras.

Imagine there is a window in the middle of your forehead. Shut the window, close the curtains. There is a window in both of your ears. Shut the window, close the curtains. There is a window in your throat. Shut the window, close the curtains. Now right on your heart, see the window? Now shut the window, close the curtains. And now on your back in the same spot. Shut the window, close the curtains. On your solar plexus. Shut the window, close the curtains. And on the same spot on your back. Shut the window, close the curtains. Below your belly button. Shut the window, close the curtains. And on the same spot on your back. Shut the window, close the curtains.

Good night. Have wonderful dreams. I love you and I'm proud of you being you."

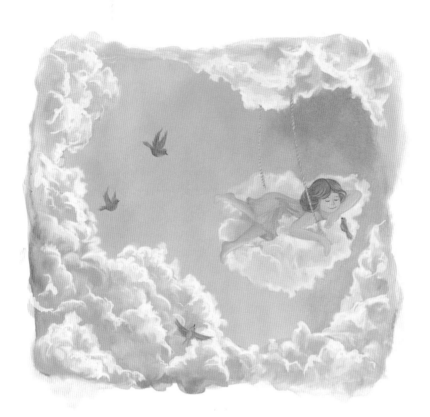

Story of
Being in the Clouds

"I want you to think of any yucky things people said or did to you today, or even things you did that you don't feel so good about. Imagine those yucky things like weeds sprouting inside you. Do you see them in your mind or in your heart or in your tummy? I want you to pluck all those ugly weeds and throw them in the bin. Now take a stick of dynamite, light it and throw that in the bin. And kaboom! All the yucky weeds are blown up, gone forever.

Now take my hand and we climb up a giant set of pink crystal stairs that reach all the way up into the sky. When we reach the top, there are two swings made out of clouds. We sit down and notice that the clouds in front of us change to a beautiful red.

Take a cup, fill it up with the red cloud and sip it. It forms a red ray from a rainbow that slides down your throat. As it goes down, you say I am...

I am..., I am..., I am... Say it three times in your head and the red ray turns to a gold seed right here.

The clouds now turn orange. Take a cup, fill it up with the orange cloud and sip it. It forms an orange ray from a rainbow that slides down your throat. As it goes down, you say I am...

I am..., I am..., I am... Say it three times in your head and the orange ray turns to a gold seed right here.

The clouds now turn yellow. Take a cup, fill it up with the yellow cloud and sip it. It forms a yellow ray from a rainbow that slides down your throat. As it goes down, you say I am...

I am..., I am..., I am... Say it three times in your head and the yellow ray turns to a gold seed right here.

The clouds now turn green. Take a cup, fill it up with the green cloud and sip it. It forms a green ray from a rainbow that slides down your throat. As it goes down, you say I am...

I am..., I am..., I am... Say it three times in your head and the green ray turns to a gold seed right here.

The clouds now turn blue. Take a cup, fill it up with the blue cloud and sip it. It forms a blue ray from a rainbow that slides down your throat. As it goes down, you say I am...

I am..., I am..., I am... Say it three times in your head and the blue ray turns to a gold seed right here.

The clouds now turn indigo. Take a cup, fill it up with the indigo cloud and sip it. It forms an indigo ray from a rainbow that slides down your throat. As it goes down, you say I am...

I am..., I am..., I am... Say it three times in your head and the indigo ray turns to a gold seed right here.

The clouds now turn violet. Take a cup, fill it up with the violet cloud and sip it. It forms a violet ray from a rainbow that slides down your throat. As it goes down, you say I am...

I am..., I am..., I am... Say it three times in your head and the violet ray turns to a gold seed right here.

Now you have seven magic seeds inside of you and to make them grow you have to pour gold light onto them. Only you have the power to do this. In the centre of your body, there is a gold light. It's right here. Pour your gold light onto the seeds. Now look and feel the seeds grow into a gold plant with branches, vines, and gold flowers. It grows all the way to the tips of your toes, fingertips and top of your head. It gets bigger and brighter. It gets so big and bright it pops outside your body.

Now you're sitting in a gold bubble. Suck the gold bubble onto your body. It forms a gold suit. Now you are spiritually safe and protected at all times. You will now have a beautiful sleep and wake up in the morning filled with happiness and ready for what the day brings.

Now I will shut your Chakras.

Imagine there is a window in the middle of your forehead. Shut the window, close the curtains. There is a window in both of your ears. Shut the window, close the curtains. There is a window in your throat. Shut the window, close the curtains. And on the same spot on the back of your throat. Shut the window, close the curtains. Now right on your heart, see the window? Now shut the window, close the curtains. And now on your back in the same spot. Shut the window, close the curtains. On your solar plexus. Shut the window, close the curtains. And on the same spot on your back. Shut the window, close the curtains. Below your belly button. Shut the window, close the curtains. And on the same spot on your back. Shut the window, close the curtains.

Good night. Have wonderful dreams. I love you and I'm proud of you being you."

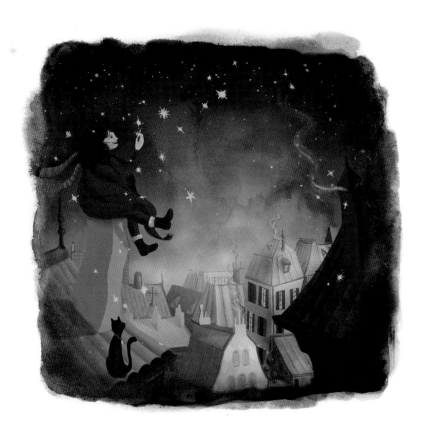

Story of the
Snowflake Stars

"I want you to think of any yucky things people said or did to you today, or even things you did that you don't feel so good about. Imagine those yucky things like weeds sprouting inside you. Do you see them in your mind or in your heart or in your tummy? I want you to pluck all those ugly weeds and throw them in the bin. Now take a stick of dynamite, light it and throw that in the bin. And kaboom! All the yucky weeds are blown up, gone forever.

Now we sit on the roof of our house/apartment and the sky is full of a million gold stars. The stars start to sparkle red and fall from the sky like snowflakes all around us.

You take a spoon and scoop up those red stars and eat them. They form a red ray from a rainbow that slides down your throat. As it goes down, you say I am...

I am..., I am..., I am... Say it three times in your head and the red ray turns to a gold seed right here.

The stars turn orange and fall from the sky. You take a spoon, scoop them up and eat them. They form an orange ray from a rainbow that slides down your throat. As it goes down, you say I am...

I am..., I am..., I am... Say it three times in your head and the orange ray turns to a gold seed right here.

The stars turn yellow and fall from the sky. You take a spoon, scoop them up and taste them. They form a yellow ray from a rainbow that slides down your throat. As it goes down, you say I am...

I am..., I am..., I am... Say it three times in your head and the yellow ray turns to a gold seed right here.

The stars turn green and fall from the sky. You take a spoon, scoop them up and taste them. They form a green ray from a rainbow that slides down your throat. As it goes down, you say I am...

I am..., I am..., I am... Say it three times in your head and the green ray turns to a gold seed right here.

The stars turn blue and fall from the sky. You take a spoon, scoop them up and taste them. They form a blue ray from a rainbow that slides down your throat. As it goes down, you say I am...

I am..., I am..., I am... Say it three times in your head and the blue ray turns to a gold seed right here.

The stars turn indigo and fall from the sky. You take a spoon, scoop them up and taste them. They form an indigo ray from a rainbow that slides down your throat. As it goes down, you say I am...

I am..., I am..., I am... Say it three times in your head and the indigo ray turns to a gold seed right here.

The stars turn violet and fall from the sky. You take a spoon, scoop them up and taste them. They form a violet ray from a rainbow that slides down your throat. As it goes down, you say I am...

I am..., I am..., I am... Say it three times in your head and the violet ray turns to a gold seed right here.

Now you need to water these magic gold seeds to make them grow and only you have the power to do this. In the centre of your being, there is a gold light. Can you see it? It's right here. I want you to put all that gold light into a watering can and pour it onto the seeds. Now look and feel the seeds grow into a gold plant with branches, vines, and gold flowers. It grows all the way to the tips of your toes, fingertips and top of your head. It gets bigger and brighter. It gets so big and bright you can't contain it in your body any more so it expands outside your body.

Now you're sitting in a gold bubble. Suck the gold bubble onto the outside of your body. It forms a gold suit. This gold suit keeps you spiritually safe and protected at all times. You will now have a beautiful sleep and wake up in the morning filled with happiness and ready for what the day brings.

Now I will shut your Chakras.

Imagine there is a window in the middle of your forehead. Shut the window, close the curtains. There is a window in both of your ears. Shut the window, close the curtains. There is a window in your throat. Shut the window, close the curtains. And on the same spot on the back of your throat. Shut the window, close the curtains. Now right on your heart, see the window? Now shut the window, close the curtains. And now on your back in the same spot. Shut the window, close the curtains. On your solar plexus. Shut the window, close the curtains. And on the same spot on your back. Shut the window, close the curtains. Below your belly button. Shut the window, close the curtains. And on the same spot on your back. Shut the window, close the curtains.

Good night. Have wonderful dreams. I love you and I'm proud of you being you."

Thank you

Evan and Ben - my awesome boys - you bring out the joy from within me. I am one proud mama and know you will grow into beautiful men just like Dad (but men who can dance!).

Mike - my gorgeous man - our love throughout my journey has only grown bigger and brighter and even if you don't understand it all I love the fact that you listen (and nod). Your support for my passions makes my heart sing even louder.

Family and friends - my peeps - you are the juice in my life vein. You keep me laughing and dancing and laughing some more. You have been there cheering me on even when I was flopping around and had no idea who I was or what I was doing.

Denise - my soul sister and book designer - we have been on this ride together for almost 20 years and seen the good, the bad and now the beautiful. You are extraordinary. Deep hugs.

Deb - my spiritual mentor - you helped me see and understand my SELF and for this I am forever grateful. Your teachings and guidance are the light behind this entire project and me.

Glynis - my fab assistant - I knew the moment we met you were going to be the best righthand woman to get things done and keep me in line. Your wonderful energy is palpable.

Fab - my lovely friend and videographer - you rock and just happen to be one of the most talented and creative photographers I have had the pleasure to work with.

Kris - my clever editor - your kind and caring manner helped me take an enormous leap into a wonderful and unknown world. You are Sleepy Magic's best friend.

Ina - my talented illustrator - Sleepy Magic has come alive with your magical illustrations. It was inspiring collaborating with such a creative mind.

Dara - my web guru- you have encapsulated what the book and what I am all about in your online creation. You made the process fun and incredibly easy.

Lauren - my talented photographer - you pulled out the beauty in me and captured my essence... I think the two wines helped.

David Cunningham - my artist friend - I know you are laughing at that title! Because of you, the Room to Read Charity (www. roomtoread.org) has come into my life. You have opened a very important door for me, my boys and the rest of the Sleepy Magic Community.

Danielle LaPorte, Marie Forleo, KC Baker, Tiphani Montgomery, Angela Raspass, Megan Dalla-Camina and Jessica Larsen - my rocking women resources - this book is here because you ladies gave me the cahoonas to make it happen. I respect each and every one of you and your brilliance that is shining upon the world.

B School hotties, The Women's Thought Leadership Society chicks, and The Best Sellers Project Babes - my social network tribes - through all of your shared triumphs and tribulations I have learned a ridiculous amount. I wish you all success in life.

The Sleepy Magic Community - my growing family - you are a gift to me. I hope by reading this little book it will open a new chapter for you and your beautiful, bold and bright children.

I am grateful. I am grateful. I am grateful.

Love+Light

Danielle Wright

Resources and reads:

Guided meditations

Deborah Beers Meditations - *(www.deborahbeers.com)*
Silva Meditations - App *(www.silvamethod.com)*
Paul McKenna, I Can Make You Sleep - App
(www.paulmckenna.com)
Oprah and Deepaks 21-Day Meditation MP3 download -
(chopracentermeditation.com)
Gabrielle Bernstein Meditations, free online sign up - *(gabbyb.tv)*
Barry Goldstein Meditation Music CD or MP3 download -
(www.barrygoldsteinmusic.com)

Books

Mind Calm: The Modern-Day Meditation - Sandy C. Newbigging
(www.sandynewbigging.com)
Breaking the Habit of Being Yourself - How to Lose your Mind and
Create a New One - Dr. Joe Dispenza *(www.drjoedispenza.com)*
The Alchemist - Paulo Coelho *(www.paulocoelho.com)*
Defy Gravity: Healing Beyond the Bounds of Reason -
Caroline Myss *(www.myss.com)*
Chakras for Beginners: How to Balance Chakras, Strengthen Aura
and Radiate Energy - Victoria Lane
The Art of Extreme Self-Care - Cheryl Richardson
(www.cherylrichardson.com)
The Desire Map: A Guide to Creating Goals with Soul -
Danielle LaPorte *(www.daniellelaporte.com)*
Women's Bodies, Women's Wisdom - Dr. Christiane Northrup
(www.drnorthrup.com)

E-Squared: Nine Do-It-Yourself Energy Experiments that Prove your Thoughts Create your Reality - Pam Grout *(www.pamgrout.com)*

The Book of Awakening - Mark Nepo *(www.marknepo.com)*

The Biology of Belief: Unleashing the Power of Consciousness, Matter & Miracles - Bruce H. Lipton *(www.brucelipton.com)*

You Can Heal Your Life - Louise L. Hay *(www.louisehay.com)*

How to Stop Worrying and Start Living - Dale Carnegie *(www.dalecarnegie.com)*

The Untethered Soul: The Journey Beyond Yourself - Michael A. Singer *(www.untetheredsoul.com)*

The Law of Attraction: The Basics of the Teaching of Abraham - Esther Hicks *(www.abraham-hicks.com)*

A New Earth: Create a Better Life - Eckhart Tolle *(www.eckharttolle.com)*

The Seven Spiritual Laws Of Success - Deepak Chopra *(www.deepakchopra.com)*

A Return to Love - Marianne Williamson *(www.marianne.com)*

Wishes Fullfilled: Mastering the Art of Manifesting - Dr. Wayne Dyer *(www.drwaynedyer.com)*

The Lighterworker's Way - Doreen Virtue *(www.angeltherapy.com)*

Notes of inspiration

I am inspired	I am cool
I am calm	I am real
I am trustworthy	I am fearless
I am compassionate	I am inspirational
I am kind	I am important
I am fit	I am excited
I am accepted	I am bright
I am joyful	I am smart
I am whole	I am open
I am fabulous	I am loving
I am a rockstar	I am courageous
I am focused	I am extraordinary
I am free	I am wonderful
I am brave	I am a free spirit
I am fast	I am brilliant
I am patient	I am determined
I am me	I am energized
I am bold	I am excited
I am intelligent	I am friendly
I am fun	I am grateful
I am super-duper	I am magical
I am caring	I am open-hearted
I am awesome	I am relaxed

I am love

I am giving

I am empowered

I am alive

I am generous

I am creative

I am honest

I am healthy

I am successful

I am funny

I am positive

I am divine

I am protected

I am peaceful

I am unique

I am cherished

I am valued

I am centred

I am clear

I am secure

I am safe

I am sweet

I am thankful

I am thrilled

I am treasured

I am warm

I am cuddly

I am fantastic

I am epic

I am helpful

I am handsome

I am beautiful

I am amazing

I am superb

I am sensational

I am excellent

I am incredible

I am outstanding

I am marvellous

I am phenomenal

I am dynamite

I am remarkable

I am forgiving

I am gentle

I am interesting

I am strong

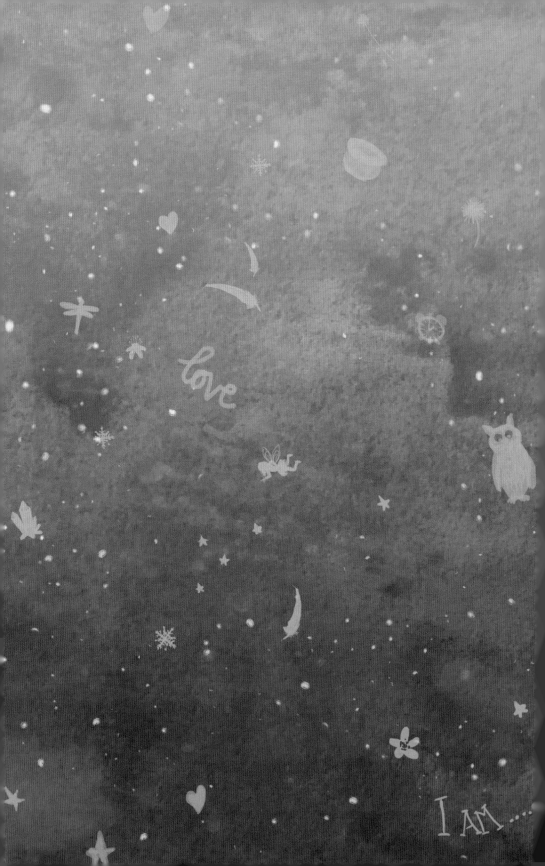

love

I AM....